Healthy Eating for Wellness

Destroy Fat, Restore Your Metabolism, and Live Healthier

By

Marlon Bowen

Disclaimer

Copyright © by Marlon Bowen 2023. All rights reserved.

Before this document is duplicated or reproduced in any manner, the publisher's consent must be gained.

Therefore, the content within can neither be stored electronically, transferred nor kept in the database. Neither in part or full can the document be copied, scanned, faxed or retrained without the approval from the publisher or creator.

Table of contents

Introduction

A healthy lifestyle starts with proper nutrition, which is essential to preserving overall wellness. The food we eat gives our bodies the energy and nutrients they require to function at their peak, repair and regenerate cells, and keep a healthy weight. But many people battle with bad food that can result in weight gain, a sluggish metabolism, and a variety of other health issues in today's fast-paced society where convenience frequently takes precedence over nutrition.

Healthy eating for wellbeing has gained popularity in recent years as a way to enhance wellness and fend off chronic diseases through the consumption of a well-balanced diet. With this strategy, the significance of eating whole, minimally processed meals are emphasized, along with the need to watch portion sizes and stay away from potentially dangerous components like trans fats.

In this context, one of the primary objectives of healthy eating is to eliminate extra fat and reestablish a balanced metabolism, which can aid in lowering the risk of obesity,heart disease, diabetes, and other chronic illnesses. People can acquire a healthier weight and enhance their general health by paying close attention to the suggestions in this book.This article addresses the fundamentals of a balanced diet for wellbeing, including the contribution of particular foods to health promotion and useful advice for establishing healthy eating practices. Healthy eating can lay a strong basis for accomplishing your wellness objectives, whether they be to lose weight, increase energy, or just feel better in your skin.

Chapter 1

Astounding Science about Fats: the Terrible, the in-between, and the better

Why are polyunsaturated and monounsaturated fats healthy, trans fats unhealthy, and saturated fats in the middle?

Fat was a four-letter word for a long time. We were advised to avoid it as much as we could in our meals. We started eating low-fat meals. But despite this, we did not become healthier as a result of the change, likely because we reduced both dangerous and beneficial fats.

Isn't fat unhealthy for you, you might be wondering? Nonetheless, your body needs some dietary fat. It is a significant source of energy. It aids in several vitamins and minerals absorption. Fat is required to construct cell membranes, each cell's essential outer layer, and the sheaths that enclose neurons. It is necessary for inflammation, muscular contraction, and blood clotting. Some fats are better than others in terms of long-term health. Examples of healthy fats are Monounsaturated and polyunsaturated fats. Trans fats made in factories are included in the bad ones. Saturated fats are in the middle of the spectrum.

The chemical composition of all fats is the same: a chain of carbon atoms joined to hydrogen atoms. The amount of hydrogen atoms joined to the carbon atoms and the length and shape of the carbon chain are what distinguish one fat from another. Insignificant structural variations result in significant variations in form and function.

Terrible trans fats

The trans fat variety of dietary fat is the worst sort. It is a result of a procedure called hydrogenation, which solidifies good oils and keeps them from becoming bad. There is no safe level of trans fat consumption, and they have no established health benefits. Trans fats were mostly present in solid margarine and vegetable shortening around the turn of the 20th century. As food producers discovered new applications for partly hydrogenated vegetable oils, they began to appear in everything from commercial cookies and pastries to fast-food French fries. Trans fats are now forbidden in the United States and many other countries.

Consuming foods high in trans fats raises blood levels of bad LDL cholesterol and lowers levels of good HDL cholesterol.

Inflammation brought on by trans fats has been related to diabetes, heart disease, stroke, and other chronic illnesses. They increase the risk of type 2 diabetes by inducing insulin resistance. Trans fats can be unhealthy in any proportion; for every 2% of daily calories ingested in trans fat, the risk of heart disease increases by 23%.

In-between saturated fats

Saturated fat: what is it? Red meat, full milk and other dairy products, cheese, coconut oil, and many commercially produced baked goods and other foods are common sources of saturated fat. The number of hydrogen atoms that surround each carbon atom is referred to as being "saturated" in this context. The carbon atom chain is saturated with hydrogen atoms, holding as many of them as is physically possible.

Can saturated fat harm your health? A diet high in saturated fats can raise total cholesterol and shift the scales in favor of more dangerous LDL cholesterol, which causes blockages to form in arteries throughout the body, including those that provide blood to the heart. Because of this, the majority of nutritionists advise keeping saturated fat intake to under 10% of daily calories.

The relationship between saturated fat and heart disease has been clouded by a few recent studies. According to a meta-analysis of 21 studies, there is insufficient data to conclude that saturated fat raises the risk of heart disease, while switching to polyunsaturated fats may lower that risk. The recommendations were narrowed slightly by two additional significant studies, which concluded that the best strategy for lowering the risk of heart disease is to replace saturated fat with polyunsaturated fats like vegetable oils or high-fiber carbohydrates, whereas replacing saturated fat with highly processed carbohydrates may have the opposite effect.

Better monounsaturated and polyunsaturated fats

Fish, nuts, seeds, and vegetables are the main sources of healthy fats. They differ from saturated fats in that their carbon chains are less tightly bound with hydrogen atoms. At standard temperature, healthy fats are liquid, not solid. The two main types of healthy fats are monounsaturated and polyunsaturated.

Monounsaturated fats.

There is only one carbon-to-carbon double bond in monounsaturated fats. As a result, it has a bend at the double bond and two fewer hydrogen atoms than saturated fat. Monounsaturated fats are kept liquid at normal temperature by this structure. Olive oil, peanut oil, canola oil, avocados, the majority of nuts, high-oleic safflower and sunflower oils, and peanut butter are all excellent sources of monounsaturated and polyunsaturated fats.

The Seven Countries Study conducted in the 1960s helped scientists realize that monounsaturated fat may have health benefits. It showed that despite eating a high-fat diet, people in Greece and other Mediterranean countries had a low rate of heart disease. Yet, they did not consume the saturated animal fat that is typical in nations with a higher prevalence of heart disease. That was olive oil, which includes mostly monounsaturated fat. This discovery led to a rise in interest in olive oil and the

"Mediterranean diet," which is now seen as a healthy eating option. The National Academy of Medicine advises replacing saturated and trans fats with monounsaturated fats as much as feasible, coupled with polyunsaturated fats, even though there is no recommended daily intake for them.

Polyunsaturated fats.

Very likely, you're utilizing polyunsaturated fat when you add liquid cooking oil to a skillet. Common examples include corn oil, sunflower oil, and safflower oil. Essential fats include polyunsaturated fats. This means that even if your body cannot produce them, they are necessary for regular bodily processes. Hence, you must consume food to obtain them. Cell membranes and the coating of nerves are made of polyunsaturated lipids. They are required for inflammation, muscular contraction, and blood clotting.

The carbon chain of a polyunsaturated lipid has two or more double bonds. Polyunsaturated fats primarily fall into two categories: omega-3 fatty acids and omega-6 fatty acids. The numbers represent the separation between the first double bond and the start of the carbon chain. Both have advantages for your health. Consuming polyunsaturated fats rather than saturated fats or carbs that have undergone extensive processing lowers dangerous LDL cholesterol and enhances the lipid profile. Triglycerides are also reduced by it. Fatty fish like salmon, mackerel, sardines, flaxseeds, walnuts, canola oil, and unhydrogenated soybean oil are excellent sources of omega-3 fatty acids. Safflower, soybean, sunflower, walnut, and corn oils are examples of vegetable oils that are high in linoleic acid and other omega-6 fatty acids.

Chapter 2

Restore Your Body Metabolism

Certain foods contain nutrients that boost metabolism or the rate at which the body burns calories, among other things. Some foods that may increase metabolism include eggs, flaxseed, lentils, and chili peppers.
People who increase their metabolic rate may be able to lose weight and reduce their risk of obesity and related health problems.

Egg

protein-rich foods are excellent for increasing metabolism. Eggs are high in protein, with each large, hard-boiled egg containing 6.29 grams (g), making them an excellent choice for those looking to boost their metabolism. Because protein requires more energy to digest than fats or carbohydrates, it is one of the most effective nutrients for increasing metabolic rate. This energy expenditure is referred to as the thermic effect of food (TEF) or diet-induced thermogenesis by scientists (DIT).

Flaxseeds

Flaxseeds are seeds high in protein, vitamins, and other essential nutrients. Flaxseeds are considered a "functional food" by some, which means they are consumed for their health benefits. Eating flaxseeds may help improve metabolic syndrome, a group of conditions that contribute to diabetes, obesity, and cardiovascular disease. Flaxseeds boost metabolism, which is likely due to their high fiber and protein content, as well as essential omega-3 fats, antioxidants, and other nutrients. Flaxseed fiber ferments in the gut, improving the bacterial profile. This process promotes metabolic health and may help prevent obesity.

Flaxseeds and their nutrients aid in the treatment or prevention of the following conditions: arthritis, autoimmune diseases, cancer, cardiovascular disease, diabetes, neurological disorders, and osteoporosis.

Lentils

Lentils are another functional meal that can help with metabolic syndrome. Eating lentils and other legumes, such as beans and peas, can help prevent and treat metabolic syndrome. Lentils, which are high in protein, may help boost metabolism. They also have enough fiber to feed the healthy bacteria in the intestines.

Chili peppers

Spicy meals with fresh or dried chili peppers can boost metabolism and give you a sense of fullness. Capsaicin, a chemical found in peppers, is responsible for these and other health advantages. Consuming capsaicin increases metabolic rate and can help with weight management in other ways by boosting the pace at which the body consumes fat and decreasing appetite. Capsaicin may also help treat illnesses including rheumatoid arthritis and Alzheimer's disease by reducing pain and inflammation, acting as an anticancer agent, and providing antioxidant effects.

Ginger

Adding ginger to meals could improve body warmth and metabolic rate, and help reduce appetite. The spice may aid to lower body weight and fasting glucose levels while raising high-density lipoprotein (HDL), or "good" cholesterol. Ginger has anti-inflammatory effects and may aid in nausea reduction during pregnancy and after chemotherapy treatment.

Coffee

Because of the caffeine concentration, coffee can accelerate metabolism. Caffeine use stimulates energy expenditure and can result in a higher metabolism. However, it is critical to keep total consumption in mind. Decaffeinated coffee does not provide the same metabolic boost. Additionally, adding cream or sugar raises the calorie content, which may counteract the caffeine's favorable benefits on metabolism.

Brazilian nuts

Brazil nuts are high in selenium, a mineral that is necessary for metabolism, reproduction, and immunological function. They also contain protein and healthy fats, which help individuals feel full.

Selenium is particularly crucial for the thyroid gland, which regulates the metabolic activity and produces a number of critical hormones. However, people should avoid consuming too many nuts because this can lead to selenium poisoning. Brazil nuts can help healthy people lower their cholesterol levels. A high amount of cholesterol is a sign of the metabolic syndrome.

Broccoli

Broccoli contains a chemical called glucoraphanin, which may help with metabolism. Glucoraphanin helps to "retune" metabolism, lower blood fat levels, and minimize the risk of a variety of age-related disorders. Broccoli and other cruciferous vegetables may also help to prevent or halt the progression of some cancers.

Vegetables with Dark, Leafy Green Leaves

Because of their high iron content, spinach, kale, and other leafy green vegetables may help improve metabolism. Iron is a mineral that is required for metabolism, growth, and development.

Chapter 3

Create your Healthy Eating plan

A healthy eating plan is much like a puzzle that needs to be put together. As with any puzzle, you could be left scratching your head at first, unsure of how you will manage to fit all the various jigsaw pieces together. You will learn about tools and guidelines in this area that will help you develop a thorough understanding of the nutrients that are best for you. The following are the things you must do;

Examine your Current Food Consumption
Examining your present food consumption, which involves obtaining information about your regular eating patterns, is the first step in developing a healthy eating plan. A food

journal is an ideal instrument for this task. You can keep track of the meals, snacks, and liquids you consume throughout the day by keeping a food journal. It is a good idea to keep a food journal for a few days in a row because your daily food intake will vary, giving you a more accurate picture of your present eating patterns. The quantities of all the meals and beverages you consume, as well as the cooking techniques utilized, should be recorded in a thorough food journal. Was the food, for instance, boiled, fried, or cooked in butter?

Check for Six accepted Diet-planning principles & (DRI)

Adequacy, Balance, Calorie Control, Nutrient Density, Moderation, and Variety are the six acknowledged diet-planning concepts. Dietary Reference Intakes are a collection of reference values for the intake of nutrients and energy that are used to plan and assess the diets of healthy people.

Look for your Nutritional Demand

Once you have that piece of the puzzle in place, you can move on to the next step, which entails using proven tools and guides created to assist you in identifying your nutritional demand. Dietary Reference Intakes (DRIs), which are guidelines for the proper nutritional consumption that healthy persons require in order to maintain their health, are predetermined. DRIs are designed to be appropriate for people of all genders and ages because your nutritional needs vary depending on your gender, age, and life circumstances like pregnancy.

Construct your Eating Schedule

The DRIs and six generally accepted diet-planning principles provide information on the amounts of each nutrient you should consume as well as suggestions for good eating practices, but they do not list the specific items that satisfy these dietary requirements. As a result, you require the following puzzle piece, which explains how to create your eating plan and choose the specific items you will eat. There are nutritional guidelines based on dietary guidelines that might assist you with this component of your healthy eating plan. These meal guidelines are straightforward visual representations that classify foods into five categories: vegetables, fruits, grains, proteins, and dairy. They then quickly display the ideal ratios from each category that make up a balanced diet.

Monitor Your Development

Your healthy eating program is almost finished; the last step is to gauge your success. It's crucial to arrange routine visits with your doctor to keep an eye on health indicators like your blood pressure, weight, and blood chemistry if you want to ensure that your plan is fulfilling your needs.

You now have all the ingredients to put together a nutritious eating schedule that will keep your health on track for happiness.

Chapter 4

Building a Healthy Eating Plan

One of the most crucial things you can do to safeguard your health is to eat a nutritious diet. In fact, lifestyle choices and behaviors like eating a nutritious diet and exercising regularly can prevent up to 80% of early heart disease and stroke.

A nutritious diet can minimize your risk of heart disease and stroke by lowering your blood pressure, managing your weight, lowering your cholesterol, and improving your blood sugar levels.

The following items must be included in your meal plan:

Consume a Lot of Fruit and Vegetables

One of the most remarkable dietary practices is this. Fruit and vegetables are abundant in nutrients (vitamins, minerals,antioxidants and fiber) and help you maintain a healthy weight by making you feel satisfied for longer periods of time. At every meal and snack, put fruit and vegetables on half of your plate.

Select Whole Grain Products

Brown or wild rice, quinoa, oatmeal, whole-wheat bread, crackers, and hulled barley are examples of whole-grain foods. Foods made from whole grains contain fiber, protein, and B vitamins to keep you feeling fuller for longer. Instead of processed grains like white bread and pasta, choose whole-grain options. Half of your plate should be made up of whole-grain items.

Eat Protein-rich Food

Nuts, legumes, seeds, fortified soy beverages, fish, shellfish,poultry, lean red meats, eggs, including wild game, low-fat milk, low-fat yogurts, low-fat kefir, and low-fat and low-sodium cheeses are examples of foods high in protein. Building and nourishing bones, muscles, and skin both require protein.

Reduce the intake of highly and Ultra-processed Meals

Foods that have undergone extensive processing also referred to as ultra-processed foods, differ significantly from their original food sources. Important nutrients including vitamins, minerals, and fiber are frequently lost during processing while salt and sugar are added. White rice, fast food, hot dogs, chips, cookies, frozen pizzas, and white bread are a few examples of processed foods. Some minimally processed foods, those that have been marginally altered but contain few industrially produced additives are acceptable. Almost all of the nutrients in minimally processed foods are still present. Vegetables, bagged salad, frozen fruit, eggs, milk, cheese, flour, brown rice, oil, and dry herbs are some examples. When we suggest that you avoid processed foods, we are not referring to these minimally processed foods.

Choose to Drink only Water

Without adding calories to the diet, water improves hydration and supports health. Energy drinks, fruit drinks, 100% fruit juice, soft drinks, and flavored coffees are among the sugary beverages that have a lot of sugar but little to no nutritional benefit. Without realizing it, it is simple to consume empty calories, which causes weight gain. Avoid fruit juice, even if it is made entirely of fruit. Fruit juice contains some of the same vitamins and minerals as fruit, but it also contains more sugar and less fiber. Fruits should be consumed, not drunk. Coffee, tea, unsweetened lower-fat milk, and previously boiled water can all be used to relieve your thirst when there is no safe drinking water available.

Chapter 5

How to Stop Emotional Eating

How does emotional eating work?
Emotional eating is the practice of consuming food to satisfy emotional rather than gastrointestinal demands. Sadly, emotional eating doesn't address emotional issues. Actually, it usually makes you feel worse. Following that, the underlying emotional issue persists, and you also feel guilty for overindulging.

Emotional Eating Cycle

It's not necessarily bad to use food as a pick-me-up, a reward, or a celebration every once in a while, but when it becomes your main emotional coping mechanism and your first reaction is to open the refrigerator whenever you feel stressed, upset, angry, lonely, exhausted, or bored, you enter a dangerous cycle where the underlying cause of your feelings or issue is never addressed. Food can never satisfy emotional hunger. Even while eating may feel nice at the moment, the emotions that caused the cravings are still present. And a lot of times the extra calories you just ate make you feel worse than you did before. You blame yourself for making a mistake and lacking greater determination.

Contrasting Bodily Hunger with Emotional hunger

You must first learn to differentiate between emotional and physical hunger in order to escape the cycle of emotional eating. This may be more difficult than it appears, particularly if you frequently use food to cope with your emotions. Because emotional hunger may be so strong, it's simple to confuse it with actual hunger. However, there are signs you can look for to differentiate between physical and emotional hunger. A sudden emotional hunger strikes. It comes at you suddenly and feels urgent and overwhelming.

On the other hand, physical hunger develops more gradually. The need to eat does not feel as intense or call for immediate gratification. Specific comfort foods are craved during emotional hunger. When you are physically hungry, practically anything, even healthful foods like vegetables sounds appetizing. However, emotional hunger yearns for fast meals or sugary snacks that give an immediate high. Nothing else will do when you feel the need for pizza or cheesecake. Mindless eating is frequently a result of emotional hunger. Before you know it, you've consumed a whole pint of ice cream or a whole bag of chips without really paying attention to what you're doing or truly enjoying it. You are usually more conscious of your actions when you are eating to satisfy physical hunger. Being full does not satisfy emotional hunger. You frequently eat until you're uncomfortable because you keep wanting more and more food. Contrarily, there is no necessity to sate physical hunger. When you have a full stomach, you feel satisfied.

The stomach does not contain emotional hunger. Instead of experiencing a growling stomach or a twinge in your stomach, you experience hunger as a mental longing. You are concentrating on particular tastes, textures, and odors. The result of emotional hunger is frequently regret, remorse, or humiliation. Since you are simply providing for your body's necessities when you eat to quell physical hunger, you are unlikely to experience any remorse or shame. If you feel bad after eating, it's probably because you know in your heart that you are not eating for nutrition.

Common Causes of Emotional Eating

Stress

The more stress is out of control in your life, the more likely you are to turn to food for emotional comfort. Have you ever observed how stress makes you hungry? It's not just in your head. Chronic stress, which is so common in our chaotic environment, causes your body to create high quantities of the stress hormone cortisol, which increases your desires for fried, salty, and sweet foods, which give you an energy and pleasure boost.

Burying Feelings

Anger, fear, despair, anxiety, loneliness, resentment, and shame are just a few of the unpleasant emotions that eating might help temporarily "stuff down" or suppress. You can avoid the uncomfortable emotions you'd prefer not to feel by numbing yourself with food.

Boredom or Empty Sensations

Do you ever use food as a means to pass the time, get rid of boredom, or fill a vacuum in your life? Food is a means to keep your tongue and your time busy while you're feeling empty and unfulfilled. It gives you energy in the present and takes your mind off underlying emotions of emptiness and discontent with your existence.

Childhood Customs

Consider your early memories of eating. Did your parents treat you to ice cream for good behavior, take you out for pizza when you received good grades, or give you sweets when you were depressed? These behaviors frequently persist throughout maturity. Or you can be motivated by fond recollections of baking and eating cookies with your mom or grilling hamburgers in the garden with your dad.

Social Factors

Having a meal with others is a terrific way to decompress, but it can also result in overeating. Simply because the food is available or because everyone else is eating, it is simple to overindulge. Additionally, social anxiety may cause you to overeat. Or perhaps you are encouraged to overeat by your friends or family, and it is simpler to fit in.

Put an End to Emotional Eating

At least a few of the previous descriptions likely contained you. Finding your unique triggers is the first step in stopping emotional eating. What situations, position, or emotions cause you to turn to food for comfort? The majority of emotional eating is associated with negative emotions, but it can also be brought on by pleasurable sensations, like rewarding yourself for reaching a goal or enjoying a special occasion.

Keep Track of your Emotional Eating

Keeping a food and mood diary is one of the best ways to spot the trends behind your emotional eating. Take a moment to consider what caused the urge each time you overeat or feel forced to grab your comfort meal. If you watch careful, you will discover a distressing incident that started the cycle of emotional eating. Record everything in your diet and mood journal: what you ate or wanted to eat, what irritated you, how you felt prior to eating, how you felt throughout your meal, and how you felt afterward. You'll start to notice a pattern after some time. Perhaps you always overindulge after hanging out with a judgmental friend. Or maybe you overeat when you have a deadline or when you go to family gatherings. The next stage is to find healthier ways to fuel your feelings after you've determined what triggers your emotional eating.

Look for Alternative Ways to Satisfy your Emotions

You won't be able to regulate your eating behaviors for very long if you don't know how to manage your emotions without using food. Because diets offer reasonable nutritional advice that can only be followed if you have conscious control over your eating habits, they frequently fail. When emotions take over and demand food as immediate gratification, the process fails. You must discover alternative strategies to satisfy your emotions if you want to stop emotional eating. Understanding the cycle of emotional eating or even your own triggers is a crucial first step, but it is not sufficient. You need emotional satiation sources other than food that you can use.

A Substitute for Emotional Eating

Call a friend who always cheers you up, plays with your dog or cat, or gazes at a treasured photo or object if you are feeling down or lonely. If you're feeling tense, move it out by dancing to your favorite tune, squeezing a stress ball, or going for a quick stroll. When you're feeling worn out, treat yourself to a nice cup of tea, a bath, some scented candles, or a warm blanket. If you're bored, pass the time by reading a good book, watching a comedy special, going for a walk, or engaging in anything you find enjoyable, such as woodworking, playing the guitar, shooting hoops, scrapbooking, etc.

Chapter 6

Recipes and Meal Plans

A recipe is a written guide that describes how to make a particular dish or meal. Recipes often include a list of the necessary materials as well as detailed preparation instructions, including cooking times and temperatures. Simple, quick dinners to elaborate, multi-step feasts requiring expert cooking techniques can all be found in recipes. On the other side, a meal plan is a schedule of what to eat and when. A meal plan can be altered to accommodate particular nutritional requirements or objectives, such as weight loss or muscle growth. Meal plans can be made for a week or longer and often include breakfast, lunch, supper, and snacks.

There are a few important considerations to bear in mind while making a meal plan

Set a Target
Decide what your meal plan will help you accomplish. Are you attempting to eat healthier, get more muscle, or just lose weight?

Analyze your Calorie Requirements
The answer will vary depending on your age, gender, weight, and amount of activity. To calculate how many calories you need each day, utilize an online calculator.

Pick Foods that Support your Objectives
You might need to prioritize particular food groups, such as lean proteins or complex carbohydrates, depending on your objective.

Think Ahead.

Spend some time organizing your meals for the coming week. By doing this, you may save time and guarantee that you have all the necessary components on hand.

Be Adaptable

Don't be hesitant to modify your eating plan as necessary. When life happens, you might need to make quick adjustments.

There are a few different places you can utilize to find recipes for your food plan

Cookbooks

There are innumerable cookbooks available that are devoted to various cuisines, nutritional requirements, and cooking techniques.

Online Recipe Repositories

There are vast recipe databases that you can browse through on websites like Allrecipes, Epicurious, and Food Network.

Instagram and Pinterest

Are wonderful platforms for finding recipe writers and food bloggers who post their favorite dishes.

Apps

Mealime, Yummly, and Cookpad are just a few of the applications that may be used to find recipes.

Conclusion

In conclusion, a healthy lifestyle can help people attain and maintain optimal health, and a balanced diet for wellness is a crucial part of a healthy lifestyle. Individuals can eliminate extra fat and reestablish a healthy metabolism, which will enhance their general health and well-being, by adopting a balanced and nutritious diet rich in whole, minimally processed foods and avoiding toxic substances. People can adopt long-lasting dietary and lifestyle adjustments that support good health and stave off chronic diseases by including certain nutrients and useful advice for healthy eating. These adjustments could involve eating more fruits and vegetables, consuming less processed food and sugar, and being mindful of portion sizes.

Even while adopting substantial lifestyle and dietary changes can be difficult, the advantages of healthy eating for wellbeing make it well worth the effort. Healthy eating is an important part of leading a satisfying and vibrant life because it can help people have more energy, a better mood, and live longer.

www.ingramcontent.com/pod-product-compliance
Lightning Source LLC
Chambersburg PA
CBHW061532250726
48657CB00005B/2191